DIABETIC DESSERTS COOKBOOK 2024

Easy and Delicious Recipes to Satisfy Sweet Cravings While Managing Blood Sugar Levels

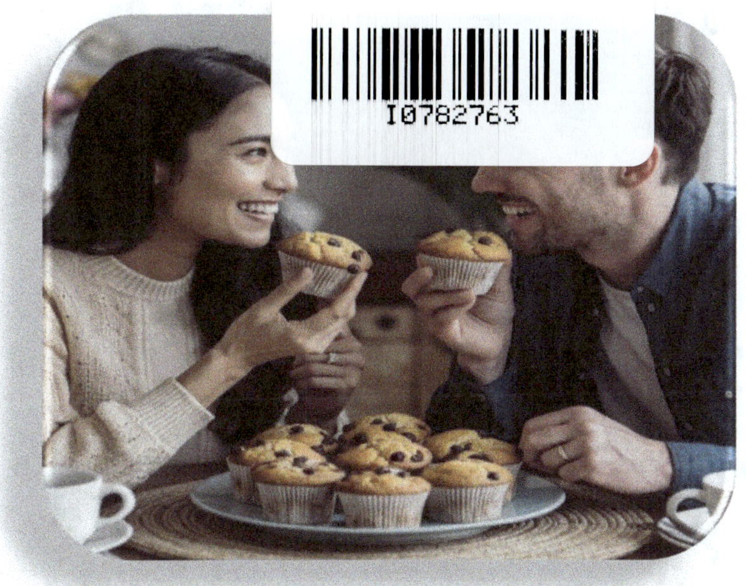

Susana Haley

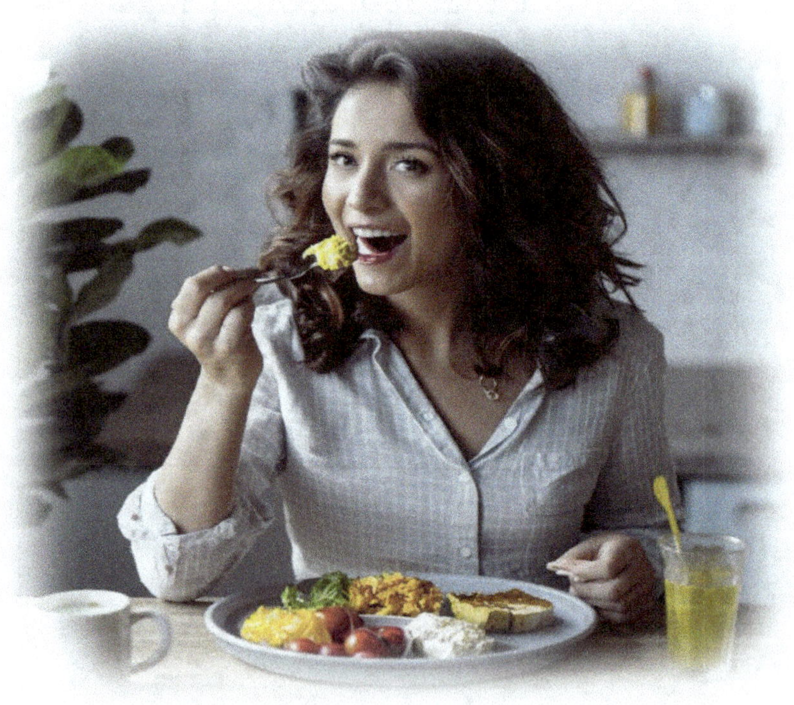

TABLE OF CONTENTS

INTRODUCTION

Welcome to the Diabetic Desserts Cookbook 2024! If you're holding this book, chances are you're on a quest for delectable treats that won't send your blood sugar on a rollercoaster ride. Well, you've landed in the right place! In these pages, you'll discover a treasure trove of easy and delicious recipes designed specifically with your sweet cravings and blood sugar levels in mind.

But first, let's address the elephant in the room – diabetes. It's a condition that affects millions worldwide, requiring diligent management and mindful choices, especially when it comes to food. However, being diabetic doesn't mean bidding farewell to the joy of indulging in desserts. Far from it! With the right ingredients, techniques, and a sprinkle of creativity, you can whip up mouthwatering treats that satisfy your sweet tooth while keeping your blood sugar in check.

In this cookbook, we've curated a collection of recipes that are not only diabetic-friendly but also bursting with flavor and texture. Whether you're craving fruity delights, comforting breads, irresistible muffins, or classic cookies, we've got you covered. Each recipe has been meticulously crafted and tested to ensure it meets our standards of taste, healthiness, and ease of preparation.

Now, you might be wondering, "What sets this cookbook apart from the rest?" Well, aside from the delicious recipes, we've packed this book with invaluable insights and tips to help you become a master of diabetic desserts. From understanding the basics of diabetes and blood sugar management to learning how to navigate the world of sugar substitutes and alternative flours, we've got all the bases covered. You'll also find practical advice on portion control, flavor balancing, and baking techniques to elevate your dessert game.

But wait, there's more! We believe that enjoying desserts should be a guilt-free experience, which is why we've included nutritional information for each recipe. Armed with this knowledge, you can make informed choices that align with your dietary needs and health goals. Plus, with our handy portion control tips, you can indulge in your favorite treats without worrying about sugar spikes.

As you embark on this culinary journey with us, remember that moderation is key. While these desserts are designed to be diabetic-friendly, it's essential to enjoy them as part of a balanced diet and active lifestyle. With that said, don't be afraid to treat yourself occasionally – after all, life is too short to deprive yourself of the simple pleasures.

So, whether you're a seasoned baker looking for new inspiration or a newbie in the kitchen eager to impress, the Diabetic Desserts Cookbook 2024 is your go-to guide for sweet satisfaction without the sugar overload. Get ready to tantalize your taste buds, nourish your body, and embrace the joy of guilt-free indulgence. Happy baking!

CHAPTER 1

Understanding Diabetes and Its Management

In today's world, diabetes has become increasingly prevalent, affecting millions of individuals globally. But what exactly is diabetes? In simple terms, diabetes is a chronic condition characterized by elevated levels of glucose (sugar) in the blood. This occurs either because the body doesn't produce enough insulin or because the cells don't respond properly to the insulin that is produced.

There are several types of diabetes, each with its own unique characteristics and management strategies. The most common types include type 1 diabetes, type 2 diabetes, and gestational diabetes.

Type 1 diabetes, often diagnosed in childhood or adolescence, is an autoimmune condition in which the body's immune system attacks and destroys the insulin-producing cells in the pancreas. As a result, individuals with type 1 diabetes require lifelong insulin therapy to regulate their blood sugar levels.

Type 2 diabetes, on the other hand, is more prevalent and typically develops later in life, although it is increasingly being diagnosed in younger individuals due to lifestyle factors such as poor diet and lack of exercise. In type 2 diabetes, the body either becomes resistant to the effects of insulin or doesn't produce enough insulin to maintain normal blood sugar levels. This type of diabetes can often be managed through lifestyle modifications, including diet, exercise, and sometimes medication.

Gestational diabetes occurs during pregnancy and affects approximately 10% of pregnant women. It is characterized by high blood sugar levels that develop or are first recognized during pregnancy. While gestational diabetes usually resolves after giving birth, it increases the risk of developing type 2 diabetes later in life for both the mother and child.

Regardless of the type of diabetes, managing blood sugar levels is crucial for preventing complications and maintaining overall health. This involves a combination of lifestyle modifications, medication, and regular monitoring.

One of the cornerstones of diabetes management is controlling blood sugar through diet. The foods we eat directly impact our blood sugar levels, so it's essential to make healthy choices that help keep glucose levels within a target range. A balanced diet rich in whole grains, lean proteins, fruits, vegetables, and healthy fats can help stabilize blood sugar levels and promote overall well-being.

In addition to diet, regular exercise plays a key role in diabetes management. Physical activity helps improve insulin sensitivity, allowing cells to better utilize glucose for energy. It also helps with weight management and reduces the risk of cardiovascular complications associated with diabetes. Most days of the week, try to get in at least 30 minutes of moderate-intensity activity, such cycling, brisk walking, or swimming.

Monitoring blood sugar levels is another essential aspect of diabetes management. This involves regularly checking blood sugar levels using a glucometer and keeping track of the results. Monitoring allows individuals to see how their lifestyle choices, such as diet and exercise, affect their blood sugar levels and helps identify patterns over time. It also enables healthcare providers to make informed decisions about treatment and medication adjustments.

For some individuals with diabetes, medication may be necessary to help control blood sugar levels. This may include oral medications that help the body use insulin more effectively or injectable insulin therapy to replace or supplement the body's insulin production. It's essential to work closely with a healthcare provider to determine the most appropriate treatment plan based on individual needs and goals.

In conclusion, understanding diabetes and its management is essential for anyone living with this chronic condition. By making healthy lifestyle choices, including following a balanced diet, staying active, monitoring blood sugar levels, and taking medications as prescribed, individuals with diabetes can lead fulfilling lives while minimizing the risk of complications. With dedication and support from healthcare providers, it is possible to successfully manage diabetes and maintain overall health and well-being.

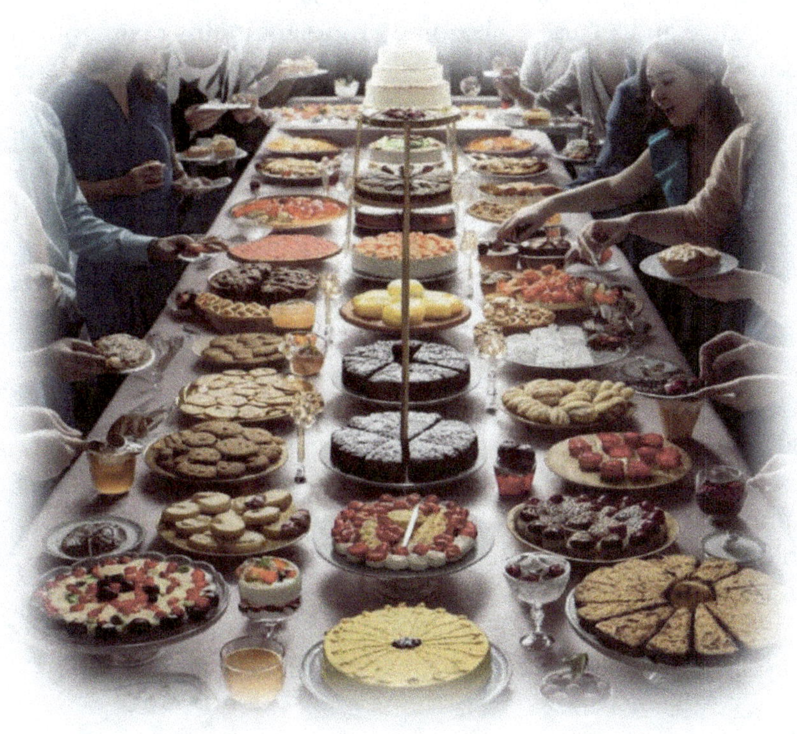

CHAPTER 2

Mastering Diabetic Desserts

In the world of diabetic desserts, mastering the art of creating delicious treats while keeping blood sugar levels in check is both a science and an art. To become proficient in this realm, one must understand the principles of diabetic-friendly baking, including the role of carbohydrates, the use of sugar substitutes, selecting the right ingredients, mastering baking techniques, and practicing portion control and moderation.

Understanding Carbohydrates and Sugar Substitutes

Carbohydrates play a significant role in blood sugar management, as they are broken down into glucose during digestion. For individuals with diabetes, it's crucial to be mindful of the types and amounts of carbohydrates consumed, as they can directly impact blood sugar levels. When creating diabetic-friendly desserts, opt for complex carbohydrates found in whole grains, fruits, and vegetables, which are digested more slowly and have less of an impact on blood sugar compared to refined carbohydrates.

In addition to carbohydrates, sweeteners are a key consideration in diabetic desserts. Traditional sugar can cause sharp spikes in blood sugar levels, making it unsuitable for individuals with diabetes. Fortunately, there are a variety of sugar substitutes available that provide sweetness without the glycemic impact. Common sugar substitutes include stevia, erythritol, monk fruit, and xylitol, each with its own unique flavor profile and sweetness intensity. Experiment with different sugar substitutes to find the ones that best suit your taste preferences and baking needs.

Selecting Ingredients for Diabetic-Friendly Desserts

When it comes to selecting ingredients for diabetic-friendly desserts, focus on whole, nutrient-dense foods that provide flavor, texture, and sweetness without the need for excessive sugar or carbohydrates. Incorporate plenty of fresh fruits, such as berries, apples, and citrus fruits, which add natural sweetness and fiber to desserts. Whole grains, such as oats, quinoa, and almond flour, can be used as alternatives to refined flours, providing complex carbohydrates and additional nutrients.

In addition to fruits and whole grains, consider incorporating healthy fats, such as nuts, seeds, and avocado, into your desserts. Not only do these fats add richness and flavor, but they also help slow down the absorption of carbohydrates, preventing rapid spikes in blood sugar levels. Experiment with different nut and seed butters, such as almond butter or tahini, to add depth and creaminess to your recipes.

Techniques for Baking with Alternative Flours

Baking with alternative flours, such as almond flour, coconut flour, and oat flour, requires a slightly different approach than traditional baking. These flours have different textures and absorbency levels, so it's essential to adjust your recipes accordingly. When substituting alternative flours for traditional flour, start by using smaller amounts and gradually increase as needed until you achieve the desired consistency.

In addition to adjusting flour quantities, consider adding binding agents, such as eggs or flaxseed meal, to help hold your baked goods together. This is especially important when using gluten-free flours, which lack the elasticity of wheat flour. Experiment with different combinations of flours and binding agents to find the ones that work best for your recipes.

Balancing Flavors and Textures in Diabetic Desserts

Creating diabetic-friendly desserts is not just about managing blood sugar levels – it's also about creating treats that are delicious and satisfying to eat. To achieve this, focus on balancing flavors and textures in your recipes. Incorporate a variety of sweet, sour, salty, and savory elements to create complexity and depth of flavor. For example, add a splash of citrus juice or zest to brighten up a dessert, or sprinkle a pinch of sea salt to enhance sweetness and contrast.

In addition to balancing flavors, pay attention to textures when creating diabetic desserts. Incorporate crunchy nuts or seeds, creamy nut butters, and chewy dried fruits to add interest and variety to your recipes. Experiment with different textures to create desserts that are not only delicious but also enjoyable to eat.

Portion Control and Moderation

While it's tempting to indulge in large portions of your favorite desserts, practicing portion control is essential for managing blood sugar levels and maintaining overall health. Instead of serving oversized portions, focus on serving smaller, more manageable portions that satisfy your sweet tooth without overloading your system with sugar and carbohydrates.

One way to practice portion control is to use smaller serving dishes and utensils when serving desserts. This creates the illusion of larger portions while actually reducing the amount of food consumed. Another strategy is to pre-portion desserts into single servings, making it easier to enjoy treats in moderation.

In addition to portion control, practicing moderation is key when it comes to enjoying diabetic desserts. Instead of indulging in sweets every day, save them for special occasions or as occasional treats. By savoring desserts in moderation, you can satisfy your sweet cravings without compromising your blood sugar management goals.

In conclusion, mastering diabetic desserts requires a combination of knowledge, skill, and creativity. By understanding the principles of diabetic-friendly baking, including carbohydrate management, ingredient selection, baking techniques, flavor balancing, and portion control, you can create delicious treats that satisfy your sweet cravings while keeping your blood sugar levels in check. With practice and experimentation, you can become a master of diabetic desserts and enjoy sweet satisfaction without the guilt.

CHAPTER 3

Diabetic Fruity Desserts

Fruits are nature's candy, packed with natural sweetness and a host of vitamins, minerals, and antioxidants. In this chapter, we'll explore five delightful recipes that celebrate the vibrant flavors of fruits while keeping blood sugar levels in check. From creamy cheesecakes to refreshing sherbets and decadent cupcakes, these diabetic-friendly fruity desserts are sure to satisfy your sweet cravings without compromising your health.

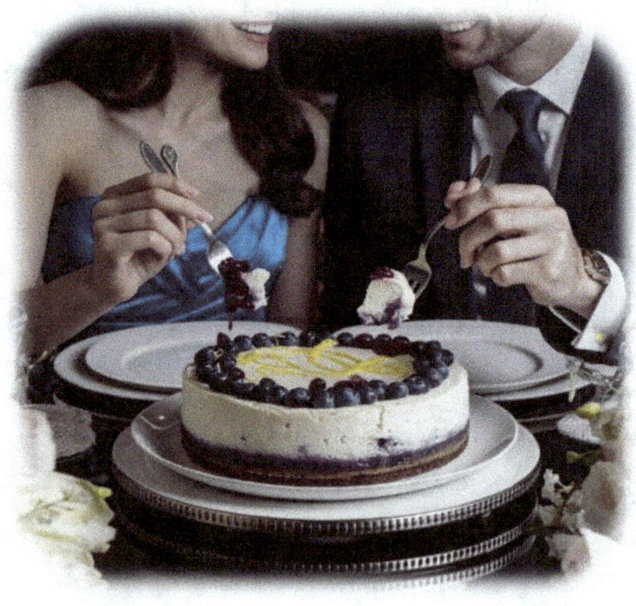

BLUEBERRY AND LEMON CHEESECAKE

Preparation Time: *20 minutes*   ***Servings:*** *8*

Ingredients:

- *1 1/2 cups almond flour*
- *1/4 cup melted coconut oil*
- *1/4 cup erythritol or preferred sugar substitute*
- *16 oz cream cheese, softened*
- 1/2 cup Greek yogurt
- 1/4 cup lemon juice
- 1 tsp lemon zest
- 1/2 cup fresh blueberries

Instructions:

- *Preheat your oven to 350°F (175°C). Grease a 9-inch springform pan.*
- *In a bowl, combine almond flour, melted coconut oil, and erythritol. To form the crust, press the mixture firmly into the bottom of the prepared pan.*
- *In another bowl, beat cream cheese until smooth. Add Greek yogurt, lemon juice, and lemon zest, and beat until well combined.*
- *Gently fold in the fresh blueberries. Over the pan's crust, pour the mixture.*
- *Bake for 30-35 minutes, or until the edges are set but the center is still slightly jiggly.*
- *Before serving, let the cheesecake cool fully and then place it in the refrigerator for at least four hours or overnight.*

PEACHY HOMEMADE SHERBET

| **Preparation Time:** *10 minutes + freezing time* | **Servings:** *4* |

Ingredients:

- *4 ripe peaches, peeled and pitted*
- *1/4 cup unsweetened almond milk*
- 2 tbsp honey or preferred sweetener
- 1 tsp vanilla extract
- 1/4 tsp lemon juice

Instructions:

- *Cut the peaches into chunks and place them in a blender or food processor.*
- *Add almond milk, honey, vanilla extract, and lemon juice to the blender.*
- *Blend until smooth and creamy.*
- *Transfer the blend into an ice cream machine and process it in accordance with the manufacturer's guidelines, often churning it for 20 to 25 minutes.*
- *Transfer the sherbet to a freezer-safe container and freeze for at least 2 hours before serving.*

LAYERED PINEAPPLE CHERRY SQUARES

Preparation Time: *15 minutes*   ***Servings:*** *9*

Ingredients:

- *1 cup almond flour*
- *1/4 cup melted coconut oil*
- *1/4 cup erythritol or preferred sugar substitute*
- *8 oz cream cheese, softened*
- 1/4 cup powdered erythritol
- 1 tsp vanilla extract
- 1 cup diced pineapple, drained
- 1 cup fresh cherries, pitted and halved

Instructions:

- *Preheat your oven to 350°F (175°C). Grease an 8x8-inch baking dish.*
- *In a bowl, combine almond flour, melted coconut oil, and erythritol. Forming the crust, press mixture into bottom of prepared baking dish.*
- *In another bowl, beat cream cheese until smooth. Add powdered erythritol and vanilla extract, and beat until well combined.*
- *Spread the cream cheese mixture evenly over the crust in the baking dish.*
- *Arrange diced pineapple and cherry halves on top of the cream cheese layer.*
- *Bake for twenty to twenty-five minutes, or until the sides are browned.*
- *Allow the squares to cool completely before slicing into servings.*

BERRY CHOCOLATE CUPCAKES

Preparation Time: *15 minutes*   ***Servings:*** *12*

Ingredients:

- *1 1/2 cups almond flour*
- *1/4 cup cocoa powder*
- *1/4 cup erythritol or preferred sugar substitute*
- *1 tsp baking powder*
- *1/4 tsp salt*
- *2 eggs*
- *1/4 cup melted coconut oil*
- 1/4 cup unsweetened almond milk
- 1 tsp vanilla extract
- One cup of mixed berries, including blueberries, strawberries, and raspberries

Instructions:

- *Preheat your oven to 350°F (175°C). Line a muffin tin with paper liners.*
- *In a bowl, whisk together almond flour, cocoa powder, erythritol, baking powder, and salt.*
- *In another bowl, beat eggs, melted coconut oil, almond milk, and vanilla extract until well combined.*
- *Gradually add the dry ingredients to the wet ingredients, mixing until smooth.*
- *Fold in the mixed berries.*
- *Using a spatula, evenly distribute the batter into the muffin cups.*
- *Put the toothpick in the center and bake for twenty to twenty-five minutes, or until it comes out clean.*
- *Allow the cupcakes to cool completely before serving.*

NICOLE'S BANANA PUDDING PIE

| **Preparation Time:** 20 minutes | **Servings:** 8 |

Ingredients:

- 1 1/2 cups almond flour
- 1/4 cup melted coconut oil
- 1/4 cup erythritol or preferred sugar substitute
- 2 ripe bananas, mashed
- 1/4 cup unsweetened almond milk
- 2 eggs
- 1 tsp vanilla extract
- 1/4 tsp cinnamon
- 1/4 tsp nutmeg
- 1/4 tsp salt
- 1/4 cup chopped walnuts (optional)

Instructions:

- Preheat your oven to 350°F (175°C). Grease a 9-inch pie dish.
- In a bowl, combine almond flour, melted coconut oil, and erythritol. Press the mixture into the bottom of the prepared pie dish to form the crust.
- In another bowl, whisk together mashed bananas, almond milk, eggs, vanilla extract, cinnamon, nutmeg, and salt until well combined.
- Pour the banana mixture over the crust in the pie dish.
- Sprinkle chopped walnuts evenly over the top, if desired.
- Bake for 25-30 minutes, or until the filling is set and the edges are golden brown.
- Allow the pie to cool completely before slicing into servings.

BERRYLICIOUS PARFAIT

| **Preparation Time:** 10 minutes | **Servings:** 2 |

Ingredients:

- *1 cup Greek yogurt*
- *One cup of mixed berries, including blueberries, raspberries, and strawberries*
- 1/4 cup of finely chopped nuts, like walnuts or almonds
- 2 tbsp honey or preferred sweetener
- Fresh mint leaves for garnish (optional)

Instructions:

- *In a bowl, mix Greek yogurt and honey until well combined.*
- *In serving glasses or bowls, layer Greek yogurt mixture, mixed berries, and chopped nuts.*
- *Layers can be repeated until all of the cups or bowls are filled.*
- *Garnish with fresh mint leaves, if desired.*
- *Transfer to the refrigerator until ready to serve, or serve immediately.*

ORANGE CREAM PIE

Preparation Time: *20 minutes + chilling time*

Servings: *8*

Ingredients:

- *1 pre-made pie crust (store-bought or homemade)*
- *1 cup unsweetened almond milk*
- *1/2 cup freshly squeezed orange juice*
- *2 tbsp cornstarch*
- 1/4 cup honey or preferred sweetener
- 1 tsp vanilla extract
- Zest of 1 orange
- 1/2 cup whipped cream (optional)

Instructions:

- *Preheat your oven to 375°F (190°C). Bake the pre-made pie crust according to package instructions, then let it cool completely.*
- *In a saucepan, whisk together almond milk, orange juice, cornstarch, honey, vanilla extract, and orange zest over medium heat.*
- *Cook the mixture, stirring constantly, until it thickens and coats the back of a spoon, about 5-7 minutes.*
- *Pour the orange cream mixture into the cooled pie crust.*
- *Pie should be chilled for four hours or more to set.*
- *If preferred, garnish with whipped cream prior to serving.*

CRUSTLESS LEMON CREAM PIE

Preparation Time: *10 minutes + baking and chilling time*

Servings: *6*

Ingredients:

- *1 cup Greek yogurt*
- *1/2 cup freshly squeezed lemon juice*
- *Zest of 2 lemons*
- *1/4 cup honey or preferred sweetener*
- 2 tbsp cornstarch
- 1 tsp vanilla extract
- 1/2 cup whipped cream (optional)
- Lemon slices for garnish (optional)

Instructions:

- *In a bowl, whisk together Greek yogurt, lemon juice, lemon zest, honey, cornstarch, and vanilla extract until smooth.*
- *Pour the mixture into a greased pie dish or individual ramekins.*
- *Bake at 350°F (175°C) for 20-25 minutes, or until set.*
- *Before serving, let the pie cool fully and then place it in the refrigerator for at least two hours.*
- *Top with whipped cream and garnish with lemon slices, if desired.*

LIGHT & AIRY RASPBERRY-RHUBARB PIE

Preparation Time: *20 minutes + baking and cooling time*

Servings: *8*

Ingredients:

- *1 pre-made pie crust (store-bought or homemade)*
- *2 cups chopped rhubarb*
- *2 cups fresh raspberries*
- *1/4 cup honey or preferred sweetener*
- 2 tbsp cornstarch
- 1 tsp vanilla extract
- 1/2 tsp cinnamon
- 1/4 tsp nutmeg
- 1/4 cup chopped nuts (such as almonds or pecans)

Instructions:

- *Preheat your oven to 375°F (190°C). Bake the pre-made pie crust according to package instructions, then let it cool completely.*
- *In a saucepan, combine chopped rhubarb, raspberries, honey, cornstarch, vanilla extract, cinnamon, and nutmeg.*
- *For about ten to fifteen minutes, or until the fruit is tender and the sauce thickens, cook the mixture over medium heat, stirring regularly.*
- *Transfer the mixed fruit into the pie shell that has cooled.*
- *Sprinkle chopped nuts over the top.*
- *Bake for an additional 15-20 minutes, or until the nuts are toasted and the filling is bubbly.*
- *Allow the pie cool fully before cutting into slices and serving.*

PEACH MELBA 'N' CREAM TRIFLE

Preparation Time: *15 minutes*   ***Servings:*** *4*

Ingredients:

- *2 cups cubed angel food cake*
- *2 cups sliced peaches*
- *1 cup fresh raspberries*
- *1 cup Greek yogurt*
- 1/4 cup honey or preferred sweetener
- 1 tsp vanilla extract
- 1/4 cup chopped almonds or walnuts (optional)

Instructions:

- *Blend honey, vanilla extract, and Greek yogurt in a bowl until smooth.*
- *In serving glasses or bowls, layer cubed angel food cake, sliced peaches, and fresh raspberries.*
- *Spoon Greek yogurt mixture over the fruit layers.*
- *Layers can be repeated until all of the cups or bowls are packed.*
- *Garnish with chopped nuts, if desired.*
- *Serve immediately or refrigerate till you are ready to serve.*

These fruity desserts are not only delicious but also diabetic-friendly, allowing you to indulge in sweet treats without worrying about blood sugar spikes. Whether you prefer the creamy texture of parfaits, the lusciousness of pies, or the lightness of trifles, there's something for everyone in this chapter. Enjoy the natural sweetness of fruits in every bite and savor the joy of guilt-free indulgence.

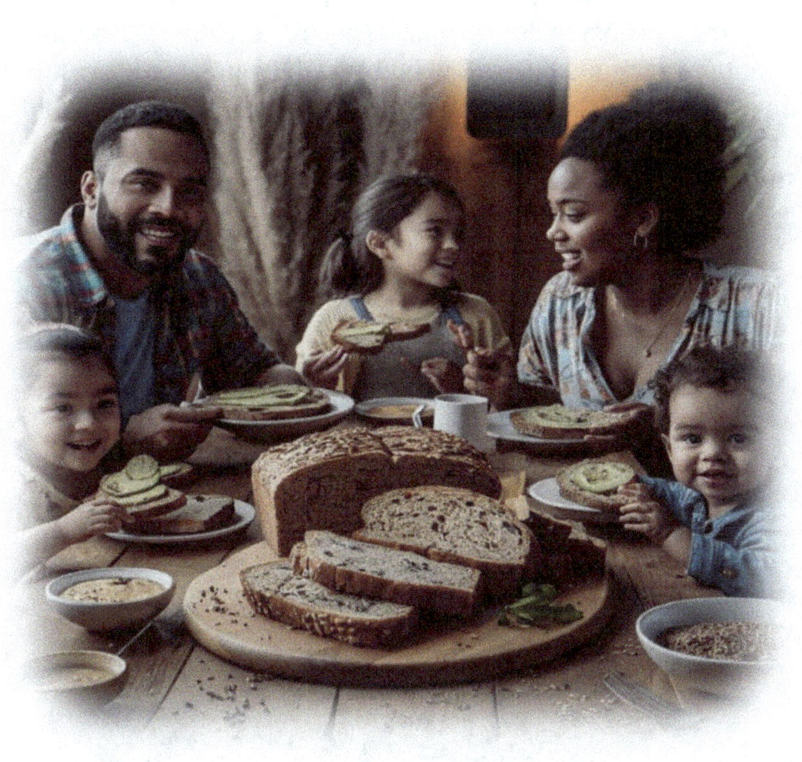

CHAPTER 4
Diabetic Bread Recipes

Bread is a staple in many diets, but for individuals managing diabetes, choosing the right type of bread is essential for maintaining blood sugar levels. In this chapter, we'll explore five diabetic-friendly bread recipes that are not only delicious but also nutritious, providing fiber, protein, and healthy fats to help stabilize blood sugar levels.

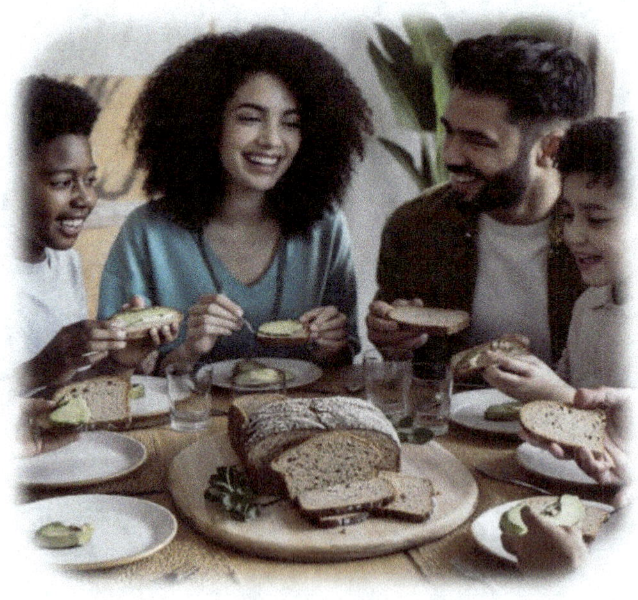

SPROUTED GRAIN BREAD

Preparation Time: *15 minutes*   **Servings:** *10*

Ingredients:

- *2 cups sprouted grain flour*
- *1/4 cup almond flour*
- *1/4 cup flaxseed meal*
- *1 tsp baking powder*
- *1/2 tsp baking soda*
- *1/2 tsp salt*
- *2 eggs*
- 1/4 cup unsweetened almond milk
- 1/4 cup olive oil
- 2 tbsp honey or preferred sweetener
- 1/4 cup chopped nuts or seeds (optional)

Instructions:

- *Preheat your oven to 350°F (175°C). Grease a loaf pan with olive oil or line it with parchment paper.*
- *In a large bowl, whisk together sprouted grain flour, almond flour, flaxseed meal, baking powder, baking soda, and salt.*
- *In another bowl, beat eggs, almond milk, olive oil, and honey until well combined.*
- *Stirring constantly, gradually incorporate the wet components into the dry ingredients until a smooth batter develops.*
- *If desired, mix with chopped nuts or seeds.*
- *Level the top of the loaf pan with a spatula after the batter has been added.*
- *Now o ahead and bake for 40 to 45 minutes or till when a toothpick put into the middle of it comes out clean*
- *After allowing the bread to cool in the pan for ten minutes, move it to a wire rack to finish cooling before slicing.*

WHOLE WHEAT FLAXSEED BREAD

Preparation Time: *15 minutes*   **Servings:** *10*

Ingredients:

- *2 cups whole wheat flour*
- *1/2 cup ground flaxseeds*
- *1 tsp baking powder*
- *1/2 tsp baking soda*
- *1/2 tsp salt*
- *2 eggs*
- *1/4 cup unsweetened almond milk*
- *1/4 cup olive oil*
- *2 tbsp honey or preferred sweetener*

Instructions:

- *Preheat your oven to 350°F (175°C). Grease a loaf pan with olive oil or line it with parchment paper.*
- *In a large bowl, whisk together whole wheat flour, ground flaxseeds, baking powder, baking soda, and salt.*
- *In another bowl, beat eggs, almond milk, olive oil, and honey until well combined.*
- *Stirring constantly, gradually incorporate the wet components into the dry ingredients until a smooth batter develops.*
- *Level the top of the loaf pan with a spatula after the batter has been added.*
- *Bake for 45–50 minutes, or until a toothpick inserted into the middle of the loaf comes out clean.*
- *After allowing the bread to cool in the pan for ten minutes, move it to a wire rack to finish cooling before slicing.*

ALMOND FLOUR BREAD

Preparation Time: *15 minutes*   **Servings:** *10*

Ingredients:

- *2 cups almond flour*
- *1/4 cup flaxseed meal*
- *1 tsp baking powder*
- *1/2 tsp baking soda*
- *1/2 tsp salt*
- *4 eggs*
- *1/4 cup unsweetened almond milk*
- *1/4 cup olive oil*
- *1 tbsp apple cider vinegar*

Instructions:

- *Preheat your oven to 350°F (175°C). Grease a loaf pan with olive oil or line it with parchment paper.*
- *In a large bowl, whisk together almond flour, flaxseed meal, baking powder, baking soda, and salt.*
- *In another bowl, beat eggs, almond milk, olive oil, and apple cider vinegar until well combined.*
- *Stirring constantly, gradually mix in the wet components until a smooth batter emerges.*
- *Using a spatula, level the top of the batter after pouring it into the prepared loaf pan.*
- *A toothpick inserted into the center should come out clean after 40 to 45 minutes of baking.*
- *Before slicing, allow the bread to sit in the pan for ten minutes before moving it to a wire rack to cool entirely.*

OATMEAL BREAD

Preparation Time: *15 minutes*	**Servings:** *10*

Ingredients:

- *2 cups rolled oats*
- *1 cup oat flour*
- *1/4 cup flaxseed meal*
- *1 tsp baking powder*
- *1/2 tsp baking soda*
- *1/2 tsp salt*
- *2 eggs*
- *1/4 cup unsweetened almond milk*
- *1/4 cup olive oil*
- *2 tbsp honey or preferred sweetener*

Instructions:

- *Preheat your oven to 350°F (175°C). Grease a loaf pan with olive oil or line it with parchment paper.*
- *In a food processor or blender, pulse rolled oats until finely ground to make oat flour.*
- *In a large bowl, whisk together oat flour, rolled oats, flaxseed meal, baking powder, baking soda, and salt.*
- *In another bowl, beat eggs, almond milk, olive oil, and honey until well combined.*
- *Stirring constantly, gradually mix in the wet components until a smooth batter emerges.*
- *Using a spatula, level the top of the batter after pouring it into the prepared loaf pan.*
- *A toothpick inserted into the center should come out clean after 40 to 45 minutes of baking.*
- *Before slicing, allow the bread to sit in the pan for ten minutes before moving it to a wire rack to cool entirely.*

COCONUT FLOUR FLATBREAD

Preparation Time: *15 minutes*   ***Servings:*** *6*

Ingredients:

- *1/2 cup coconut flour*
- *1/4 cup almond flour*
- *1/4 cup flaxseed meal*
- *1 tsp baking powder*
- *1/2 tsp salt*

- 4 eggs
- 1/4 cup unsweetened almond milk
- 1/4 cup olive oil

Instructions:

- *In a large bowl, whisk together coconut flour, almond flour, flaxseed meal, baking powder, and salt.*
- *In another bowl, beat eggs, almond milk, and olive oil until well combined.*
- *Stirring constantly, gradually incorporate the wet components into the dry ingredients until a smooth batter develops.*
- *A nonstick saucepan should be heated to medium heat.*
- *Transfer a generous amount of batter into the skillet, ensuring it forms a narrow ring.*
- *Cook until cooked through and golden brown, 2 to 3 minutes per side.*
- *Repeat with the remaining batter.*
- *Serve the flatbreads warm or at room temperature.*

CHIA SEED BREAD

Preparation Time: *15 minutes*   **Servings:** *10*

Ingredients:

- *1 cup almond flour*
- *1/4 cup chia seeds*
- *1/4 cup flaxseed meal*
- *1 tsp baking powder*
- 1/2 tsp salt
- 4 eggs
- 1/4 cup unsweetened almond milk
- 1/4 cup olive oil

Instructions:

- *Preheat your oven to 350°F (175°C). Grease a loaf pan with olive oil or line it with parchment paper.*
- *In a large bowl, whisk together almond flour, chia seeds, flaxseed meal, baking powder, and salt.*
- *In another bowl, beat eggs, almond milk, and olive oil until well combined.*
- *Stirring constantly, gradually mix in the wet components until a smooth batter emerges.*
- *Using a spatula, level the top of the batter after pouring it into the prepared loaf pan.*
- *A toothpick inserted into the center should come out clean after 40 to 45 minutes of baking.*
- *After allowing the bread to cool in the pan for ten minutes, move it to a wire rack to finish cooling before slicing.*

PSYLLIUM HUSK BREAD

Preparation Time: *15 minutes*   **Servings:** *10*

Ingredients:

- *1 cup almond flour*
- *1/4 cup psyllium husk powder*
- *1/4 cup flaxseed meal*
- *1 tsp baking powder*
- 1/2 tsp salt
- 4 eggs
- 1/4 cup unsweetened almond milk
- 1/4 cup olive oil

Instructions:

- *Preheat your oven to 350°F (175°C). Grease a loaf pan with olive oil or line it with parchment paper.*
- *In a large bowl, whisk together almond flour, psyllium husk powder, flaxseed meal, baking powder, and salt.*
- *In another bowl, beat eggs, almond milk, and olive oil until well combined.*
- *Stirring constantly, gradually mix in the wet components until a smooth batter emerges.*
- *Using a spatula, level the top of the batter after pouring it into the prepared loaf pan.*
- *A toothpick inserted into the middle of the loaf should come out clean after 40 to 45 minutes of baking.*
- *Before slicing, allow the bread to sit in the pan for ten minutes before moving it to a wire rack to cool entirely.*

ZUCCHINI BREAD

Preparation Time: *20 minutes*   **Servings:** *10*

Ingredients:

- *1 1/2 cups almond flour*
- *1/2 cup grated zucchini*
- *1/4 cup flaxseed meal*
- *1 tsp baking powder*
- *1/2 tsp baking soda*
- *1/2 tsp cinnamon*
- *1/4 tsp nutmeg*
- *1/4 tsp salt*

- 2 eggs
- 1/4 cup unsweetened almond milk
- 1/4 cup olive oil
- 1/4 cup honey or preferred sweetener

Instructions:

- *Preheat your oven to 350°F (175°C). Grease a loaf pan with olive oil or line it with parchment paper.*
- *Grated zucchini, almond flour, flaxseed meal, baking soda, baking powder, cinnamon, nutmeg, and salt should all be combined in a big basin.*
- *In another bowl, beat eggs, almond milk, olive oil, and honey until well combined.*
- *Stirring constantly, gradually mix in the wet components until a smooth batter emerges.*
- *Using a spatula, level the top of the batter after pouring it into the prepared loaf pan.*
- *A toothpick inserted into the middle of the loaf should come out clean after 45 to 50 minutes of baking.*
- *Before slicing, allow the bread to sit in the pan for ten minutes before moving it to a wire rack to cool entirely.*

CLOUD BREAD

Preparation Time: *10 minutes*	**Servings:** *6*

Ingredients:
- *3 eggs, separated*
- *3 tbsp cream cheese, softened*
- 1/4 tsp cream of tartar
- Pinch of salt

Instructions:
- *Preheat your oven to 300°F (150°C). Line a baking sheet with parchment paper.*
- *In a large bowl, beat egg whites with cream of tartar until stiff peaks form.*
- *In another bowl, beat egg yolks with cream cheese until smooth.*
- *Gently fold the egg yolk mixture into the egg whites until combined.*
- *Spoon the mixture onto the prepared baking sheet to form small rounds.*
- *Bake for 25-30 minutes, or until golden brown.*
- *Let the cloud bread cool on the baking sheet for 5 minutes, then transfer it to a wire rack to cool completely.*

SUNFLOWER SEED & HONEY WHEAT BREAD

| **Preparation Time:** *15 minutes* | **Servings:** *10* |

Ingredients:

- *1 1/2 cups whole wheat flour*
- *1/4 cup sunflower seeds*
- *1/4 cup flaxseed meal*
- *1 tsp baking powder*
- *1/2 tsp baking soda*
- 1/2 tsp salt
- 2 eggs
- 1/4 cup unsweetened almond milk
- 1/4 cup olive oil
- 1/4 cup honey

Instructions:

- *Preheat your oven to 350°F (175°C). Grease a loaf pan with olive oil or line it with parchment paper.*
- *In a large bowl, whisk together whole wheat flour, sunflower seeds, flaxseed meal, baking powder, baking soda, and salt.*
- *In another bowl, beat eggs, almond milk, olive oil, and honey until well combined.*
- *Stirring constantly, gradually mix in the wet components until a smooth batter emerges.*
- *Using a spatula, smooth the top of the batter after pouring it into the prepped loaf pan.*
- *A toothpick inserted into the middle of the loaf should come out clean after 40 to 45 minutes of baking.*
- *Before slicing, allow the bread to sit in the pan for ten minutes before moving it to a wire rack to cool entirely.*

These diabetic-friendly bread recipes offer a delicious alternative to traditional bread, allowing you to enjoy the comforting taste and texture of bread without worrying about blood sugar spikes.

Experiment with different ingredients and variations to find the ones that suit your taste preferences and dietary needs. Whether you prefer the nuttiness of chia seeds, the fiber-richness of psyllium husk, or the subtle sweetness of zucchini, there's something for everyone in this chapter. Enjoy these homemade bread recipes as part of a balanced diet to support your health and well-being

CHAPTER 5
Diabetic Muffin Recipes

Muffins are a delightful treat that can be enjoyed any time of day, whether as a quick breakfast, a satisfying snack, or a sweet dessert. However, for individuals managing diabetes, traditional muffin recipes loaded with refined flour and sugar can pose a challenge. In this chapter, we'll explore five diabetic-friendly muffin recipes that are not only delicious but also low in carbohydrates and sugar, making them suitable for maintaining stable blood sugar levels.

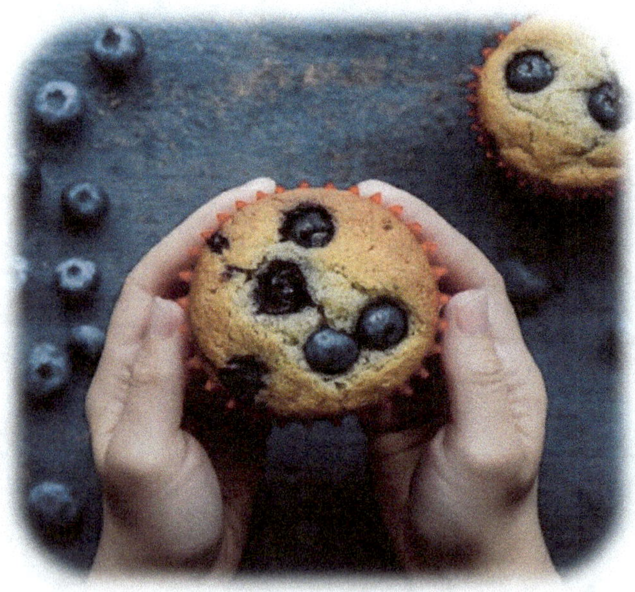

DIABETIC BLUEBERRY MUFFINS GRAIN-FREE, GLUTEN-FREE BLUEBERRY MUFFIN RECIPE

Preparation Time: *15 minutes*   ***Servings:*** *12*

Ingredients:

- *2 cups almond flour*
- *1/4 cup coconut flour*
- *1/4 cup granulated erythritol or preferred sweetener*
- *1 tsp baking powder*
- *1/2 tsp baking soda*
- *Pinch of salt*
- *3 large eggs*
- 1/4 cup unsweetened almond milk
- 1/4 cup melted coconut oil or butter
- 1 tsp vanilla extract
- 1 cup fresh or frozen blueberries

Instructions:

- *Preheat your oven to 350°F (175°C). Use paper liners or coconut oil to butter or line a muffin pan.*
- *In a large bowl, whisk together almond flour, coconut flour, erythritol, baking powder, baking soda, and salt.*
- *In another bowl, beat eggs, almond milk, melted coconut oil or butter, and vanilla extract until well combined.*
- *Stirring constantly, gradually incorporate the wet components into the dry ingredients until a smooth batter develops.*
- *Gently fold in the blueberries.*
- *Pour the batter into each muffin cup, filling it to approximately 3/4 of the way.*
- *A toothpick put into the center of the muffins should come out clean after 20 to 25 minutes of baking, or until they are golden brown.*
- *After five minutes of cooling in the pan, move the muffins to a wire rack to finish cooling before serving.*

BANANA CHOCOLATE CHIP MUFFINS

Preparation Time: 20 minutes   *Servings:* 12

Ingredients:

- *2 ripe bananas, mashed*
- *1/4 cup coconut oil, melted*
- *1/4 cup honey or preferred sweetener*
- *2 eggs*
- *1 tsp vanilla extract*
- *1 1/2 cups almond flour*
- 1/4 cup coconut flour
- 1 tsp baking powder
- 1/2 tsp baking soda
- Pinch of salt
- 1/2 cup sugar-free chocolate chips

Instructions:

- *Preheat your oven to 350°F (175°C). Use paper liners or coconut oil to butter or line a muffin pan.*
- *In a large bowl, combine mashed bananas, melted coconut oil, honey, eggs, and vanilla extract.*
- *In another bowl, whisk together almond flour, coconut flour, baking powder, baking soda, and salt.*
- *Stirring to ensure complete blending, gradually add the dry ingredients to the wet components.*
- *Fold in the sugar-free chocolate chips.*
- *Pour the batter into each muffin cup, filling it to approximately 3/4 of the way.*
- *A toothpick put into the center of the muffins should come out clean after 20 to 25 minutes of baking, or until they are golden brown.*
- *After five minutes of cooling in the pan, move the muffins to a wire rack to finish cooling before serving.*

HEALTHY ZUCCHINI MUFFINS

Preparation Time: *20 minutes*   **Servings:** *12*

Ingredients:

- *1 cup shredded zucchini*
- *1/4 cup coconut oil, melted*
- *1/4 cup honey or preferred sweetener*
- *2 eggs*
- *1 tsp vanilla extract*
- *1 1/2 cups almond flour*
- *1/4 cup coconut flour*
- 1 tsp baking powder
- 1/2 tsp baking soda
- Pinch of salt
- 1 tsp ground cinnamon
- 1/4 cup chopped walnuts or pecans (optional)

Instructions:

- *Preheat your oven to 350°F (175°C). Use paper liners or coconut oil to butter or line a muffin pan.*
- *In a large bowl, combine shredded zucchini, melted coconut oil, honey, eggs, and vanilla extract.*
- *In another bowl, whisk together almond flour, coconut flour, baking powder, baking soda, salt, and ground cinnamon.*
- *When the liquid components are fully blended, gradually add the dry ingredients and stir.*
- *Fold in the chopped walnuts or pecans, if using.*
- *Pour the batter into each muffin cup, filling it to approximately 3/4 of the way.*
- *A toothpick put into the center of the muffins should come out clean after 20 to 25 minutes of baking, or until they are golden brown.*
- *After five minutes of cooling in the pan, move the muffins to a wire rack to finish cooling before serving.*

ALMOND FLOUR BLUEBERRY MUFFINS

Preparation Time: *15 minutes*   **Servings:** *12*

Ingredients:

- *1 1/2 cups almond flour*
- *1/4 cup granulated erythritol or preferred sweetener*
- *1 tsp baking powder*
- *1/2 tsp baking soda*
- *Pinch of salt*
- 2 large eggs
- 1/4 cup unsweetened almond milk
- 1/4 cup melted coconut oil or butter
- 1 tsp vanilla extract
- 1 cup fresh or frozen blueberries

Instructions:

- *Preheat your oven to 350°F (175°C). Use paper liners or coconut oil to butter or line a muffin pan.*
- *Mix the almond flour, erythritol, baking soda, baking powder, and salt in a big basin.*
- *In another bowl, beat eggs, almond milk, melted coconut oil or butter, and vanilla extract until well combined.*
- *Stirring constantly, gradually incorporate the wet components into the dry ingredients until a smooth batter develops.*
- *Fold in the blueberries gently.*
- *Pour the batter into each muffin cup, filling it to approximately 3/4 of the way.*
- *A toothpick put into the middle of the muffins should come out clean after between twenty and twenty-five minutes of baking, or until they are golden brown.*
- *After five minutes of cooling in the pan, move the muffins to a wire rack to finish cooling before serving.*

COCONUT FLOUR MUFFINS WITH BERRIES

Preparation Time: *15 minutes*   **Servings:** *12*

Ingredients:

- *1/2 cup coconut flour*
- *1/4 cup granulated erythritol or preferred sweetener*
- *1 tsp baking powder*
- *1/2 tsp baking soda*
- *Pinch of salt*
- *4 eggs*
- *1/4 cup unsweetened almond milk*
- 1/4 cup melted coconut oil or butter
- 1 tsp vanilla extract
- One cup of mixed berries, comprising blueberries, raspberries, and strawberries

Instructions:

- *Preheat your oven to 350°F (175°C). Use paper liners or coconut oil to butter or line a muffin pan.*
- *In a large bowl, whisk together coconut flour, erythritol, baking powder, baking soda, and salt.*
- *In another bowl, beat eggs, almond milk, melted coconut oil or butter, and vanilla extract until well combined.*
- *Stirring constantly, gradually mix in the wet components until a smooth batter emerges.*
- *Gently fold in the mixed berries.*
- *Pour the batter into each muffin cup, filling it to approximately 3/4 of the way.*
- *A toothpick put into the middle of the muffins should come out clean after twenty to twenty-five minutes of baking, or until they are golden brown.*
- *After five minutes of cooling in the pan, move the muffins to a wire rack to finish cooling before serving.*

PUMPKIN PROTEIN MUFFINS

Preparation Time: *15 minutes*   ***Servings:*** *12*

Ingredients:

- *1 cup almond flour*
- *1/2 cup vanilla protein powder*
- *1 tsp baking powder*
- *1/2 tsp baking soda*
- *1 tsp ground cinnamon*
- *1/2 tsp ground nutmeg*
- *1/4 tsp ground cloves*
- *Pinch of salt*
- *1/2 cup pumpkin puree*
- 1/4 cup unsweetened almond milk
- 1/4 cup melted coconut oil or butter
- 2 eggs
- 1/4 cup granulated erythritol or preferred sweetener
- 1 tsp vanilla extract

Instructions:

- *Preheat your oven to 350°F (175°C). Use paper liners or coconut oil to butter or line a muffin pan.*
- *In a large bowl, whisk together almond flour, protein powder, baking powder, baking soda, cinnamon, nutmeg, cloves, and salt.*
- *In another bowl, combine pumpkin puree, almond milk, melted coconut oil or butter, eggs, erythritol, and vanilla extract.*
- *Add wet ingredients to dry ingredients gradually, stirring until well combined.*
- *Pour the batter into each muffin cup, filling it to approximately 3/4 of the way.*
- *A toothpick put into the middle of the muffins should come out clean after baking for 18 to 20 minutes, or until they are golden brown.*
- *After five minutes of cooling in the pan, move the muffins to a wire rack to finish cooling before serving.*

CARROT CAKE MUFFINS

Preparation Time: *20 minutes*   **Servings:** *12*

Ingredients:

- *1 cup almond flour*
- *1/4 cup coconut flour*
- *1 tsp baking powder*
- *1/2 tsp baking soda*
- *1 tsp ground cinnamon*
- *1/4 tsp ground nutmeg*
- *Pinch of salt*
- *1 cup shredded carrots*
- *1/4 cup chopped walnuts or pecans (optional)*
- 1/4 cup unsweetened applesauce
- 1/4 cup melted coconut oil or butter
- 2 eggs
- 1/4 cup granulated erythritol or preferred sweetener
- 1 tsp vanilla extract

Instructions:

- *Preheat your oven to 350°F (175°C). Use paper liners or coconut oil to butter or line a muffin pan.*
- *Mix the almond flour, coconut flour, baking soda, baking powder, nutmeg, cinnamon, and salt in a big basin.*
- *Stir in shredded carrots and chopped nuts, if using.*
- *In another bowl, combine applesauce, melted coconut oil or butter, eggs, erythritol, and vanilla extract.*
- *Gradually add the wet ingredients to the dry ingredients, stirring until well combined.*
- *Pour the batter into each muffin cup, filling it to approximately 3/4 of the way.*
- *A toothpick put into the middle of the muffins should come out clean after twenty to twenty-five minutes of baking, or until they are golden brown.*
- *After five minutes of cooling in the pan, move the muffins to a wire rack to finish cooling before serving.*

CHIA SEED MUFFINS

Preparation Time: *15 minutes*   ***Servings:*** *12*

Ingredients:

- *1 cup almond flour*
- *1/4 cup coconut flour*
- *2 tbsp chia seeds*
- *1 tsp baking powder*
- *1/2 tsp baking soda*
- *Pinch of salt*
- *1/2 cup unsweetened almond milk*
- 1/4 cup melted coconut oil or butter
- 2 eggs
- 1/4 cup granulated erythritol or preferred sweetener
- 1 tsp vanilla extract

Instructions:

- *Preheat your oven to 350°F (175°C). Use paper liners or coconut oil to butter or line a muffin pan.*
- *In a large bowl, whisk together almond flour, coconut flour, chia seeds, baking powder, baking soda, and salt.*
- *In another bowl, combine almond milk, melted coconut oil or butter, eggs, erythritol, and vanilla extract.*
- *Gradually add the wet ingredients to the dry ingredients, stirring until well combined.*
- *Pour the batter into each muffin cup, filling it to approximately 3/4 of the way.*
- *A toothpick put into the middle of the muffins should come out clean after baking for 18 to 20 minutes, or until they are golden brown.*
- *After five minutes of cooling in the pan, move the muffins to a wire rack to finish cooling before serving.*

AVOCADO BANANA MUFFINS

Ingredients:

- *1 cup almond flour*
- *1/4 cup coconut flour*
- *1 tsp baking powder*
- *1/2 tsp baking soda*
- *Pinch of salt*
- *1 ripe avocado, mashed*
- *2 ripe bananas, mashed*
- 1/4 cup melted coconut oil or butter
- 2 eggs
- 1/4 cup granulated erythritol or preferred sweetener
- 1 tsp vanilla extract

Instructions:

- *Preheat your oven to 350°F (175°C). Grease a 9-inch springform pan.*
- *In a bowl, combine almond flour, melted coconut oil, and erythritol. To form the crust, press the mixture firmly into the bottom of the prepared pan.*
- *In another bowl, beat cream cheese until smooth. Add Greek yogurt, lemon juice, and lemon zest, and beat until well combined.*
- *Gently fold in the fresh blueberries. Over the pan's crust, pour the mixture.*
- *Bake for 30-35 minutes, or until the edges are set but the center is still slightly jiggly.*
- *Before serving, let the cheesecake cool fully and then place it in the refrigerator for at least four hours or overnight.*

CHOCOLATE ALMOND FLOUR MUFFINS

Preparation Time: *20 minutes*	***Servings:*** *12*

Ingredients:

- *1 1/2 cups almond flour*
- *1/4 cup cocoa powder*
- *1 tsp baking powder*
- *1/2 tsp baking soda*
- *Pinch of salt*
- *1/4 cup melted coconut oil or butter*
- *1/4 cup unsweetened almond milk*
- 1/4 cup granulated erythritol or preferred sweetener
- 2 eggs
- 1 tsp vanilla extract
- 1/4 cup sugar-free chocolate chips

Instructions:

- *Preheat your oven to 350°F (175°C). Use paper liners or coconut oil to butter or line a muffin pan.*
- *In a large bowl, whisk together almond flour, cocoa powder, baking powder, baking soda, and salt.*
- *In another bowl, combine melted coconut oil or butter, almond milk, erythritol, eggs, and vanilla extract.*
- *Mixing thoroughly after each addition, gradually mix the wet and dry components together.*
- *Fold in the sugar-free chocolate chips.*
- *Pour the batter into each muffin cup, filling it to approximately 3/4 of the way.*
- *When a toothpick inserted into the middle of the muffins comes out clean, it's done baking; this should take about eighteen to twenty minutes.*
- *After five minutes of cooling in the pan, move the muffins to a wire rack to finish cooling before serving.*

These diabetic-friendly muffin recipes offer a delicious way to indulge in your favorite flavors while keeping your blood sugar levels in check. Whether you're in the mood for the warm spices of pumpkin, the comforting taste of carrot cake, the nutritious boost of chia seeds, the creamy richness of avocado and banana, or the decadent allure of chocolate, there's a muffin recipe here to satisfy every craving. Enjoy them as a convenient snack or a guilt-free treat any time of day.

CHAPTER 6
Diabetic Cookies Recipes

Cookies are a beloved treat that can bring joy to any occasion, whether enjoyed with a cup of tea, shared among friends, or savored as a sweet indulgence. However, for individuals managing diabetes, traditional cookie recipes loaded with refined sugar and carbohydrates can be off-limits. In this chapter, we'll explore five delicious diabetic-friendly cookie recipes that are low in sugar and carbohydrates, allowing you to satisfy your sweet tooth without compromising your health.

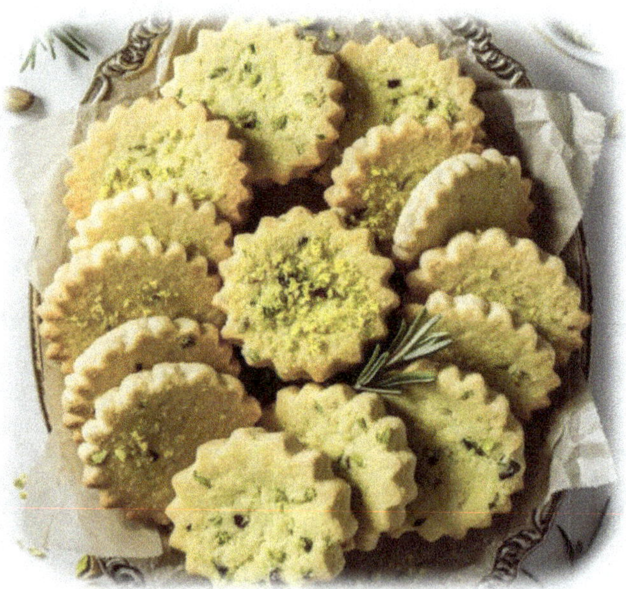

SUGAR-FREE CHOCOLATE CHIP COOKIES

Preparation Time: *20 minutes*   **Servings:** *12*

Ingredients:

- *2 cups almond flour*
- *1/4 cup granulated erythritol or preferred sweetener*
- *1/2 tsp baking soda*
- *Pinch of salt*
- 1/4 cup melted coconut oil or butter
- 1 large egg
- 1 tsp vanilla extract
- 1/2 cup sugar-free chocolate chips

Instructions:

- *Preheat your oven to 350°F (175°C). Put parchment paper on one side of a baking sheet.*
- *In a large bowl, whisk together almond flour, erythritol, baking soda, and salt.*
- *Stir in melted coconut oil or butter, egg, and vanilla extract until a dough forms.*
- *Fold in sugar-free chocolate chips.*
- *Drop tablespoon-sized portions of dough onto the prepared baking sheet, spacing them 2 inches apart.*
- *Using the back of a spoon, slightly flatten each cookie.*
- *Bake for 10-12 minutes, or until the edges are golden brown.*
- *Allow the cookies to cool on the baking sheet for 5 minutes, then transfer them to a wire rack to cool completely before serving.*

ALMOND FLOUR RASPBERRY COOKIES

Preparation Time: *25 minutes*   ***Servings:*** *12*

Ingredients:

- *2 cups almond flour*
- *1/4 cup granulated erythritol or preferred sweetener*
- *1/2 tsp baking powder*
- *Pinch of salt*
- 1/4 cup melted coconut oil or butter
- 1 large egg
- 1 tsp almond extract
- 1/2 cup fresh or frozen raspberries, chopped

Instructions:

- *Preheat your oven to 350°F (175°C). Line a baking sheet with parchment paper.*
- *Mix the erythritol, baking powder, salt, and almond flour in a big basin.*
- *Stir in melted coconut oil or butter, egg, and almond extract until a dough forms.*
- *Gently fold in chopped raspberries.*
- *Drop tablespoon-sized portions of dough onto the prepared baking sheet, spacing them 2 inches apart.*
- *Gently push each cookie down with the back of a spoon.*
- *Bake for a total of twelve to fifteen minutes, up to the point the edges are browned.*
- *Allow the cookies to cool on the baking sheet for 5 minutes, then transfer them to a wire rack to cool completely before serving.*

PISTACHIO SHORTBREAD COOKIES

Preparation Time: *40 minutes (including chilling time)*	**Servings:** *12*

Ingredients:

- *2 cups almond flour*
- *1/4 cup granulated erythritol or preferred sweetener*
- *1/2 cup shelled pistachios, finely chopped*
- Pinch of salt
- 1/4 cup melted coconut oil or butter
- 1 large egg
- 1 tsp vanilla extract

Instructions:

- *Preheat your oven to 325°F (160°C). Put parchment paper on one side of a baking sheet.*
- *In a large bowl, whisk together almond flour, erythritol, chopped pistachios, and salt.*
- *Stir in melted coconut oil or butter, egg, and vanilla extract until a dough forms.*
- *Roll the dough into a log, about 2 inches in diameter, and wrap it in plastic wrap.*
- *Chill the dough in the refrigerator for 30 minutes.*
- *Slice the chilled dough into 1/4-inch-thick rounds and place them on the prepared baking sheet.*
- *Bake until the edges begin to turn a light golden color, 12 to 15 minutes.*
- *Allow the cookies to cool on the baking sheet for 5 minutes, then transfer them to a wire rack to cool completely before serving.*

PEANUT BUTTER COOKIES

Preparation Time: *15 minutes*　　　　**Servings:** *12*

Ingredients:

- *1 cup almond flour*
- *1/2 cup natural peanut butter*
- *1 tsp vanilla extract*
- *1/4 cup granulated erythritol or preferred sweetener*
- *1 large egg*

Instructions:

- *Preheat your oven to 350°F (175°C). Put parchment paper on one side of a baking sheet.*
- *In a large bowl, mix together almond flour, peanut butter, erythritol, egg, and vanilla extract until well combined.*
- *Roll the dough into tablespoon-sized balls and place them on the prepared baking sheet.*
- *Flatten each biscuit with a fork to make a crosshatch design.*
- *Bake for 10-12 minutes, or until the edges are golden brown.*
- *Allow the cookies to cool on the baking sheet for 5 minutes, then transfer them to a wire rack to cool completely before serving.*

CHOCOLATE ALMOND TRUFFLES

Preparation Time: *15 minutes* *(plus chilling time)*	**Servings:** *12*

Ingredients:

- *1 cup almond flour*
- *1/4 cup cocoa powder*
- *1/4 cup melted coconut oil*
- *1 tsp vanilla extract*
- 1/4 cup granulated erythritol or preferred sweetener
- Unsweetened shredded coconut, for coating (optional)

Instructions:

- *In a large bowl, mix together almond flour, cocoa powder, melted coconut oil, erythritol, and vanilla extract until a dough forms.*
- *Roll the dough into tablespoon-sized balls and place them on a parchment-lined baking sheet.*
- *If desired, roll the truffles in unsweetened shredded coconut to coat.*
- *Chill the truffles in the refrigerator for at least 30 minutes before serving.*

PUMPKIN SNICKERDOODLES

Preparation Time: *25 minutes*   **Servings:** *12*

Ingredients:

- *2 cups almond flour*
- *1/4 cup granulated erythritol or preferred sweetener*
- *1 tsp baking powder*
- *1/2 tsp ground cinnamon*
- *Pinch of salt*
- *1/4 cup pumpkin puree*
- 1/4 cup melted coconut oil or butter
- 1 large egg
- 1 tsp vanilla extract
- For rolling:
- 2 tbsp granulated erythritol
- 1 tsp ground cinnamon

Instructions:

- *Preheat your oven to 350°F (175°C). Put parchment paper on one side of a baking sheet.*
- *In a large bowl, whisk together almond flour, erythritol, baking powder, cinnamon, and salt.*
- *In another bowl, mix together pumpkin puree, melted coconut oil or butter, egg, and vanilla extract until well combined.*
- *Stirring constantly, gradually mix in the wet components until a dough forms.*
- *In a small bowl, mix together granulated erythritol and ground cinnamon for rolling.*
- *Roll tablespoon-sized portions of dough into balls, then roll each ball in the cinnamon-erythritol mixture to coat.*
- *Arrange the dough balls that have been coated evenly apart on the baking sheet that has been preheated.*
- *Flatten each dough ball slightly with the back of a spoon or your fingertips.*
- *Bake for 10-12 minutes, or until the cookies are set and the edges are lightly golden.*
- *Allow the cookies to cool on the baking sheet for 5 minutes, then transfer them to a wire rack to cool completely before serving.*

EASY LOW-CARB PECAN COOKIES

Preparation Time: *20 minutes*   **Servings:** *12*

Ingredients:

- *2 cups almond flour*
- *1/4 cup granulated erythritol or preferred sweetener*
- *1/2 tsp baking soda*
- *Pinch of salt*
- 1/4 cup melted coconut oil or butter
- 1 large egg
- 1 tsp vanilla extract
- 1/2 cup chopped pecans

Instructions:

- *Preheat your oven to 350°F (175°C). Put parchment paper on one side of a baking sheet.*
- *In a large bowl, whisk together almond flour, erythritol, baking soda, and salt.*
- *In another bowl, mix together melted coconut oil or butter, egg, and vanilla extract until well combined.*
- *Stirring constantly, gradually mix in the wet components until a dough forms.*
- *Fold in chopped pecans until evenly distributed throughout the dough.*
- *Roll tablespoon-sized portions of dough into balls and place them on the prepared baking sheet, spacing them evenly apart.*
- *Flatten each dough ball slightly with the back of a spoon or your fingertips.*
- *Bake for 10-12 minutes, or until the cookies are set and the edges are lightly golden.*
- *Allow the cookies to cool on the baking sheet for 5 minutes, then transfer them to a wire rack to cool completely before serving.*

LOW-CARB ALMOND CRESCENT COOKIES

Preparation Time: *20 minutes*   ***Servings:*** *8*

Ingredients:

- *2 cups almond flour*
- *1/4 cup granulated erythritol or preferred sweetener*
- *1/2 tsp almond extract*
- *Pinch of salt*
- 1/4 cup melted coconut oil or butter
- 1 large egg
- 1/2 cup sliced almonds

Instructions:

- *Preheat your oven to 325°F (160°C). Line a baking sheet with parchment paper.*
- *In a large bowl, whisk together almond flour, erythritol, almond extract, and salt.*
- *In another bowl, mix together melted coconut oil or butter and egg until well combined.*
- *Stirring constantly, gradually mix in the wet components until a dough forms.*
- *Divide the dough into tablespoon-sized portions and shape each portion into a crescent shape.*
- *Roll each crescent-shaped cookie in sliced almonds, pressing lightly to adhere.*
- *Arrange the cookies evenly apart on the baking sheet that has been prepared.*
- *Bake for 12-15 minutes, or until the cookies are set and the edges are lightly golden.*
- *Allow the cookies to cool on the baking sheet for 5 minutes, then transfer them to a wire rack to cool completely before serving.*

COCONUT FLOUR COOKIES WITH BERRIES

Preparation Time: *25 minutes*   **Servings:** *12*

Ingredients:

- *1/2 cup coconut flour*
- *1/4 cup granulated erythritol or preferred sweetener*
- *1/2 tsp baking powder*
- *Pinch of salt*
- *1/4 cup melted coconut oil or butter*
- 1 large egg
- 1 tsp vanilla extract
- 1/2 cup mixed berries (such as strawberries, raspberries, and blueberries)

Instructions:

- *Preheat your oven to 350°F (175°C). Line a baking sheet with parchment paper.*
- *Mix the coconut flour, erythritol, baking powder, and salt in a big basin.*
- *In another bowl, mix together melted coconut oil or butter, egg, and vanilla extract until well combined.*
- *Stirring constantly, gradually mix in the wet components until a dough forms.*
- *Gently fold in mixed berries until evenly distributed throughout the dough.*
- *Roll tablespoon-sized portions of dough into balls and place them on the prepared baking sheet, spacing them evenly apart.*
- *Flatten each dough ball slightly with the back of a spoon or your fingertips.*
- *Bake for 12-15 minutes, or until the cookies are set and the edges are lightly golden.*
- *Allow the cookies to cool on the baking sheet for 5 minutes, then transfer them to a wire rack to cool completely before serving.*

ZUCCHINI CHOCOLATE CHIP COOKIES

Preparation Time: *25 minutes*   **Servings:** *12*

Ingredients:

- *1 cup almond flour*
- *1/2 cup shredded zucchini, squeezed dry*
- *1/4 cup granulated erythritol or preferred sweetener*
- *1/4 cup melted coconut oil or butter*

- 1 cup almond flour
- 1/2 cup shredded zucchini, squeezed dry
- 1/4 cup granulated erythritol or preferred sweetener
- 1/4 cup melted coconut oil or butter

Instructions:

- *Preheat your oven to 350°F (175°C). Line a baking sheet with parchment paper.*
- *In a large bowl, mix together almond flour, shredded zucchini, erythritol, melted coconut oil or butter, egg, and vanilla extract until well combined.*
- *Fold in sugar-free chocolate chips until evenly distributed throughout the dough.*
- *Drop tablespoon-sized portions of dough onto the prepared baking sheet, spacing them evenly apart.*
- *Flatten each dough ball slightly with the back of a spoon or your fingertips.*
- *Bake for 12-15 minutes, or until the cookies are set and the edges are lightly golden.*
- *Allow the cookies to cool on the baking sheet for 5 minutes, then transfer them to a wire rack to cool completely before serving.*

These diabetic-friendly cookie recipes offer a delicious way to enjoy the classic flavors of cookies without worrying about spiking your blood sugar levels. Whether you're in the mood for the warm spices of pumpkin, the nutty crunch of pecans, the delicate almond flavor of crescent cookies, the tropical taste of coconut, or the rich indulgence of chocolate chips, there's a cookie recipe here to satisfy every craving. Enjoy them as a guilt-free treat any time of day, whether on their own or paired with a hot beverage for a cozy indulgence.

CHAPTER 7

Basic Tips for Baking in the Kitchen

Baking can be a delightful and rewarding experience, especially when creating delicious desserts that are both satisfying and diabetes-friendly. In this chapter, we'll explore some essential tips and techniques to help you become a confident and successful baker in your kitchen. From understanding the necessary equipment to substituting ingredients and mastering baking techniques, these insights will empower you to create diabetic-friendly desserts that are both enjoyable and healthy.

Essential Baking Equipment for Diabetic-Friendly Desserts

Having the right tools in your kitchen can make a significant difference in your baking endeavors. Here are some essential baking equipment items you'll need to create diabetic-friendly desserts:

- ***Mixing Bowls:***
Invest in a set of mixing bowls in various sizes to accommodate different recipes. Stainless steel or glass bowls are ideal for mixing ingredients and are easy to clean.

- ***Measuring Cups and Spoons:***
Accurate measurements are crucial in baking, especially when it comes to ingredients like flour and sweeteners. Invest in a set of

measuring cups and spoons to ensure precise measurements every time.

- ***Baking Sheets:***

Baking sheets, also known as cookie sheets, are essential for baking cookies, pastries, and other treats. Opt for heavy-duty, non-stick baking sheets for even baking and easy cleanup.

- ***Muffin Tins:***

Muffin tins are versatile tools that can be used to bake muffins, cupcakes, and individual desserts. Look for non-stick muffin tins or silicone muffin molds for effortless removal of baked goods.

- ***Mixers:***

While not essential, stand mixers and hand mixers can make the process of mixing ingredients much easier and more efficient, especially for recipes that require beating eggs or creaming butter and sugar.

- ***Baking Pans:***

Invest in a variety of baking pans, including cake pans, loaf pans, and pie pans, to accommodate different types of desserts. Non-stick pans with removable bottoms are ideal for easy release of baked goods.

- ***Parchment Paper:***

Parchment paper is a baker's best friend, providing a non-stick surface for baking cookies, lining cake pans, and wrapping delicate pastries. It also makes cleanup a breeze.

- ***Cooling Racks:***

Cooling racks allow air to circulate around baked goods, preventing them from becoming soggy. Invest in a few cooling racks to cool cakes, cookies, and pastries evenly.

By having these essential baking equipment items on hand, you'll be well-prepared to tackle any diabetic-friendly dessert recipe with confidence and ease.

Substituting Ingredients in Traditional Recipes

One of the challenges of baking for individuals with diabetes is finding suitable substitutes for high-carb and high-sugar ingredients. Fortunately, there are many ingredient substitutions available that can help you create diabetic-friendly desserts without sacrificing flavor or texture. Here are some common ingredient substitutions to consider:

- ***Flour Substitutes:***
Instead of using refined wheat flour, which can cause spikes in blood sugar levels, opt for alternative flours such as almond flour, coconut flour, or oat flour. These flours are lower in carbohydrates and higher in fiber, making them suitable choices for diabetic-friendly baking.

- ***Sweeteners:***
Traditional granulated sugar can be replaced with natural sweeteners such as stevia, erythritol, or monk fruit sweetener. These sweeteners provide sweetness without affecting blood sugar levels and can be used in equal amounts as sugar in most recipes.

- ***Fruit Purees:***
Instead of using added sugars, consider using mashed bananas, unsweetened applesauce, or pureed dates to sweeten baked goods naturally. These fruit purees add moisture and sweetness to recipes without the need for additional sugar.

- ***Healthy Fats:***

Incorporating healthy fats such as coconut oil, avocado oil, or nut butters into your recipes can help balance blood sugar levels and add richness and flavor to baked goods. Replace butter or vegetable oil with these healthier alternatives for a diabetic-friendly twist.

- ***Egg Substitutes:***

For individuals with egg allergies or dietary restrictions, eggs can be replaced with alternatives such as flax eggs, chia eggs, or commercial egg replacers. These substitutes provide binding properties similar to eggs and can be used in most baking recipes.

By experimenting with these ingredient substitutions, you can create diabetic-friendly desserts that are just as delicious as their traditional counterparts while keeping your blood sugar levels in check.

Understanding Sweeteners and Their Effects

Choosing the right sweetener is essential when baking for diabetes management. While traditional sugar is off-limits for individuals with diabetes due to its high glycemic index, there are many alternative sweeteners available that can provide sweetness without causing spikes in blood sugar levels. Here are some common sweeteners and their effects:

- ***Stevia:***

The natural sweetener known as stevia is made from the leaves of the Stevia rebaudiana plant. It is intensely sweet and has zero calories and zero carbohydrates, making it an excellent choice for individuals with diabetes. Stevia is available in both liquid and powdered forms and can be used in baking and cooking.

- ***Erythritol:***

A sugar alcohol called erythritol can be found naturally in various fruits and fermented foods. It has zero calories and zero net carbohydrates, making it a popular choice for low-carb and diabetic-friendly recipes. Erythritol has a similar taste and texture to sugar and can be used in equal amounts in most recipes.

- ***Monk Fruit Sweetener:***

The monk fruit, a tiny green gourd indigenous to Southeast Asia, is the source of monk fruit sweetness. It contains natural compounds called mogrosides, which provide sweetness without raising blood sugar levels. Monk fruit sweetener is available in granulated and powdered forms and can be used as a one-to-one substitute for sugar in recipes.

- ***Xylitol:***

Xylitol is a sugar alcohol that is commonly used as a sweetener in sugar-free gum and mints. It has a sweetness similar to sugar and can be used in baking and cooking. However, it is important to note that xylitol can have a laxative effect in some individuals, so it should be used in moderation.

- ***Agave Nectar:***

Agave nectar is derived from the sap of the agave plant and is often marketed as a natural sweetener. While agave nectar has a lower glycemic index than sugar, it is still high in fructose and can raise blood sugar levels. Therefore, it should be used sparingly and in moderation.

When choosing a sweetener for diabetic-friendly baking, it's essential to consider its impact on blood sugar levels and choose options that provide sweetness without causing spikes in glucose levels. Experiment with different sweeteners to find the ones that work best for you and your dietary needs.

Baking Techniques for Optimal Results

Mastering basic baking techniques is key to creating delicious and visually appealing diabetic-friendly desserts. Whether you're whipping up a batch of cookies or baking a cake from scratch, the following techniques will help you achieve optimal results:

- ***Room Temperature Ingredients:***
Allow refrigerated ingredients such as butter, eggs, and dairy products to come to room temperature before using them in recipes. Room temperature ingredients mix more easily and evenly, resulting in smoother batters and better texture in baked goods.

- ***Proper Mixing:***
Mix dry ingredients thoroughly before adding wet ingredients to ensure even distribution of leavening agents such as baking powder and baking soda. When adding wet ingredients, mix just until combined to avoid overmixing, which can lead to tough or dense baked goods.

- ***Preheating the Oven:***
Prior to baking, always preheat your oven to the recommended temperature. By preheating, you can be sure that your baked goods will rise and cook uniformly, giving them a consistent texture and doneness.

- ***Use of Leavening Agents:***
Pay attention to the type and amount of leavening agents (such as baking powder and baking soda) called for in recipes. These ingredients help baked goods rise and achieve a light and fluffy texture. Be sure to measure leavening agents accurately to avoid over- or under-leavening.

- ***Proper Greasing and Lining:***

Grease baking pans and line them with parchment paper or silicone baking mats to prevent sticking and ensure easy removal of baked goods. This step is especially important for delicate or sticky desserts such as cakes and cookies.

- ***Even Distribution:***
When pouring batter into pans or molds, distribute it evenly to ensure that baked goods bake uniformly. Use a spatula or spoon to spread batter evenly and smooth the surface before baking.

- ***Monitoring Baking Time:***
Keep a close eye on your baked goods as they bake and adjust baking time as needed. Use a timer to prevent overbaking, which can result in dry or burnt desserts. Test for doneness by inserting a toothpick into the center of the baked item; if it comes out clean or with a few crumbs attached, it's ready.

By mastering these baking techniques, you'll be able to create diabetic-friendly desserts that are not only delicious but also visually appealing and satisfying. With practice and patience, you'll develop the skills and confidence to tackle any dessert recipe with ease.

In conclusion, mastering the art of baking for diabetes management requires a combination of the right equipment, ingredient substitutions, understanding of sweeteners, and proper baking techniques. By following the tips and techniques outlined in this chapter, you'll be well-equipped to create diabetic-friendly desserts that are both delicious and satisfying. So roll up your sleeves, preheat your oven, and get ready to indulge in guilt-free treats that won't compromise your health. Happy baking!

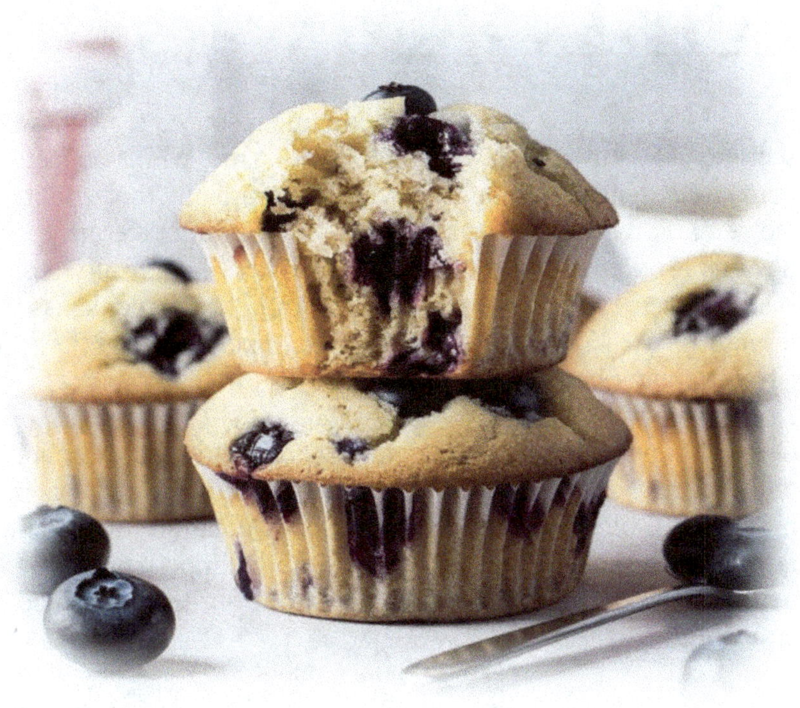

CONCLUSION

In closing, this book serves as a valuable resource for individuals seeking to indulge in delicious desserts while effectively managing their blood sugar levels. Throughout this cookbook, we've explored a wide array of easy and mouthwatering recipes designed specifically for those with diabetes. From fruity desserts to bread recipes, muffins, cookies, and more, each recipe has been thoughtfully crafted to satisfy sweet cravings without compromising health.

Our journey began with an understanding of diabetes and its management, delving into the importance of diet, exercise, monitoring blood sugar levels, and medication management. Armed with this knowledge, readers are equipped with the tools necessary to navigate their diabetes journey with confidence and empowerment.

As we ventured into mastering diabetic desserts, we explored the art of selecting ingredients, understanding carbohydrates, and utilizing sugar substitutes to create delectable treats without the guilt. Techniques for balancing flavors, textures, and portion control were highlighted, ensuring that every dessert not only delights the taste buds but also supports overall health and well-being.

Throughout the chapters dedicated to fruity desserts, bread recipes, muffins, and cookies, readers were treated to a plethora of mouthwatering options that cater to a variety of tastes and preferences. From the refreshing burst of berries to the comforting warmth of pumpkin and spices, each recipe offers a delightful escape into the world of sweet indulgence.

Moreover, the inclusion of basic tips for baking in the kitchen provides invaluable insights into essential equipment, ingredient substitutions, sweeteners, and baking techniques. Armed with these tips, readers can confidently embark on their culinary adventures, creating diabetic-friendly desserts that are both delicious and nutritious.

As we conclude our culinary journey, it's important to emphasize the versatility and creativity that diabetes-friendly cooking and baking offer. With the right ingredients and techniques, individuals with diabetes can enjoy a wide range of delectable desserts without compromising their health goals.

In the "Diabetic Desserts Cookbook 2024," we've strived to empower readers to take control of their dietary choices while still indulging in the pleasures of sweet treats. By incorporating wholesome ingredients, mindful portion control, and balanced flavors, individuals can enjoy the satisfaction of dessert without the worry of spiking blood sugar levels.

In essence, this cookbook is not just a collection of recipes; it's a celebration of delicious possibilities and a testament to the fact that living with diabetes doesn't mean sacrificing flavor or enjoyment. With a little creativity and a dash of culinary know-how, anyone can whip up diabetic-friendly desserts that are as tasty as they are wholesome.

In the end, it's not just about what you eat—it's about how you nourish your body and soul. And with the recipes and guidance found within these pages, you can enjoy the simple pleasure of dessert while keeping your blood sugar levels in check. Here's to happy, healthy indulgence, one delicious bite at a time!

THANK YOU, PAGE.

To all the readers who have embarked on this culinary journey through the "Diabetic Desserts Cookbook 2024," I extend my heartfelt gratitude. Your willingness to explore these recipes and embrace the challenge of managing blood sugar levels while satisfying sweet cravings is truly commendable.

As you savor each delectable bite and discover the joy of creating diabetes-friendly desserts, I hope you find inspiration and empowerment in these pages. Remember that delicious treats need not be off-limits, even with dietary restrictions. With a little creativity and the right guidance, you can indulge in the pleasures of dessert while prioritizing your health and well-being.

I invite you to continue your culinary adventures by exploring more books from the author Susana Haley. Whether you're seeking additional diabetic-friendly recipes, healthy cooking tips, or culinary inspiration, you'll find a wealth of resources waiting for you.

To access more books by Susana Haley, simply scan the QR code below or visit Amazon to discover a world of delicious possibilities. Thank you once again for joining me on this journey, and may your kitchen be filled with joy, flavor, and endless culinary delights.

Check out other books by the Author on Amazon below by scanning the QR code.

BONUS MADE FOR YOU

Dear Reader,
We're excited to inform you that your copy of the "Diabetic Desserts Cookbook 2024" includes an exclusive bonus: a meal planner and smoothie recipes! Inside, you'll find space to plan your meals for breakfast, lunch, dinner, and desserts daily from Monday till Sunday. This meal planner is designed to help you stay organized and on track with your diabetes management goals.

But that's not all! As an added bonus, you'll also gain access to delicious smoothie recipes that are perfect for a quick and nutritious snack or meal replacement. Simply scan the QR code at the end of this book to unlock a world of refreshing and healthy smoothie options.

We've included the meal planner and smoothie recipes as a bonus because we understand the importance of having a well-rounded approach to managing diabetes. By providing you with tools to plan your meals and enjoy nutritious smoothies, we hope to support you on your journey to better health and well-being.

We would love to hear your thoughts on the "Diabetic Desserts Cookbook 2024." If you've enjoyed the recipes and found the meal planner and smoothie recipes helpful, please consider leaving a kind review on Amazon. Your feedback helps us continue to improve and provide valuable resources to our readers.

Thank you for choosing our cookbook, and we hope it brings you joy and deliciousness in every bite!

Warm regards,
Susana Haley

SCAN ME

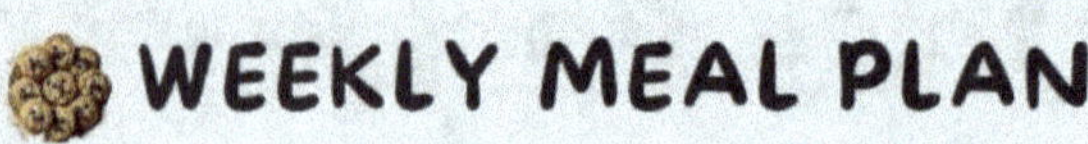

WEEKLY MEAL PLAN

MONDAY	
TUESDAY	
WEDNESDAY	
THURSDAY	
FRIDAY	
SATURDAY	
SUNDAY	

GROCERY LIST

FROM __________ TO __________

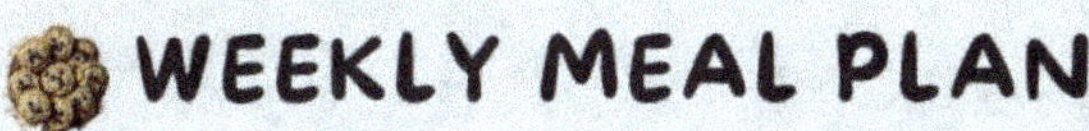

WEEKLY MEAL PLAN

MONDAY	
TUESDAY	
WEDNESDAY	
THURSDAY	
FRIDAY	
SATURDAY	
SUNDAY	

GROCERY LIST

FROM _______ TO _______

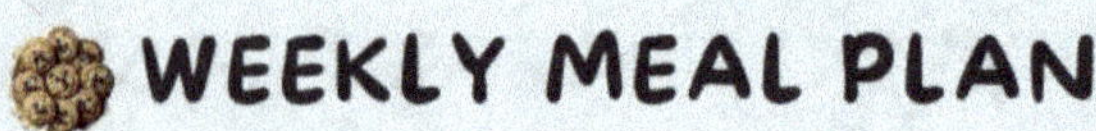

WEEKLY MEAL PLAN

MONDAY	
TUESDAY	
WEDNESDAY	
THURSDAY	
FRIDAY	
SATURDAY	
SUNDAY	

GROCERY LIST

FROM _______ TO _______

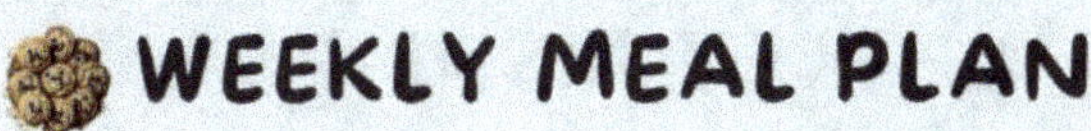

WEEKLY MEAL PLAN

MONDAY	
TUESDAY	
WEDNESDAY	
THURSDAY	
FRIDAY	
SATURDAY	
SUNDAY	

GROCERY LIST

FROM _______ TO _______

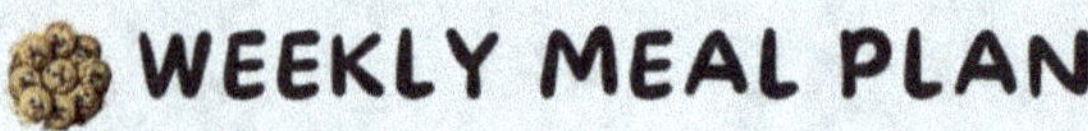

WEEKLY MEAL PLAN

MONDAY

TUESDAY

WEDNESDAY

THURSDAY

FRIDAY

SATURDAY

SUNDAY

GROCERY LIST

FROM _______ TO _______

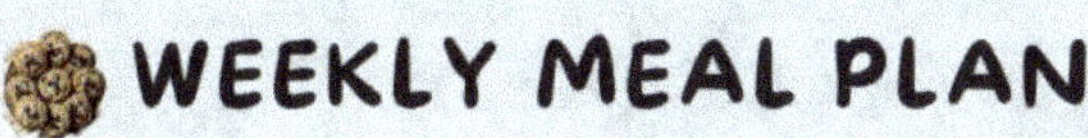 WEEKLY MEAL PLAN

MONDAY	
TUESDAY	
WEDNESDAY	
THURSDAY	
FRIDAY	
SATURDAY	
SUNDAY	

GROCERY LIST

FROM _______ TO _______

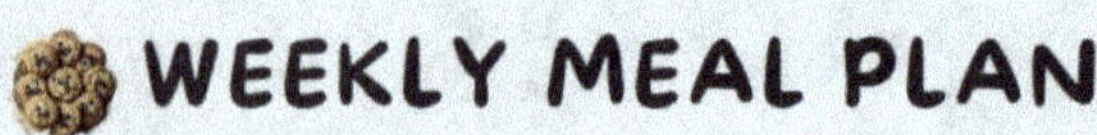

WEEKLY MEAL PLAN

MONDAY	
TUESDAY	
WEDNESDAY	
THURSDAY	
FRIDAY	
SATURDAY	
SUNDAY	

GROCERY LIST

FROM _______ TO _______

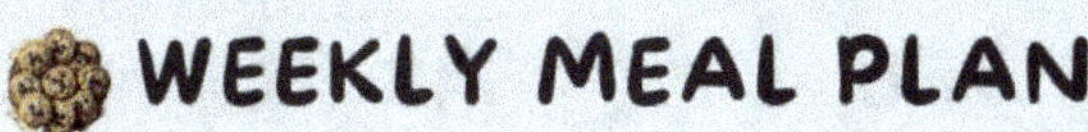

WEEKLY MEAL PLAN

MONDAY	
TUESDAY	
WEDNESDAY	
THURSDAY	
FRIDAY	
SATURDAY	
SUNDAY	

GROCERY LIST

FROM _______ TO _______

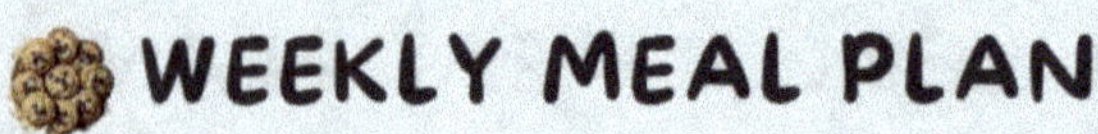

WEEKLY MEAL PLAN

	GROCERY LIST
MONDAY	
TUESDAY	
WEDNESDAY	
THURSDAY	
FRIDAY	
SATURDAY	
SUNDAY	

FROM _______ TO _______

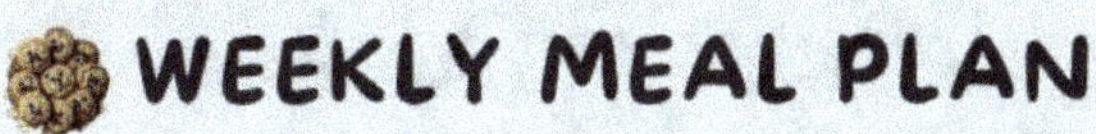 WEEKLY MEAL PLAN

MONDAY

TUESDAY

WEDNESDAY

THURSDAY

FRIDAY

SATURDAY

SUNDAY

GROCERY LIST

FROM _______ TO _______

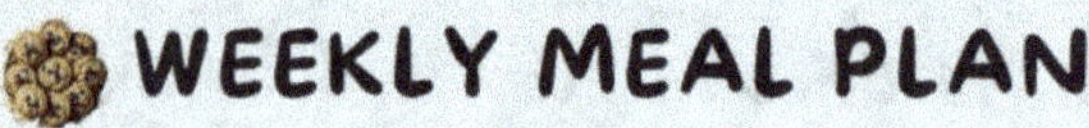

WEEKLY MEAL PLAN

MONDAY

TUESDAY

WEDNESDAY

THURSDAY

FRIDAY

SATURDAY

SUNDAY

GROCERY LIST

FROM _______ TO _______

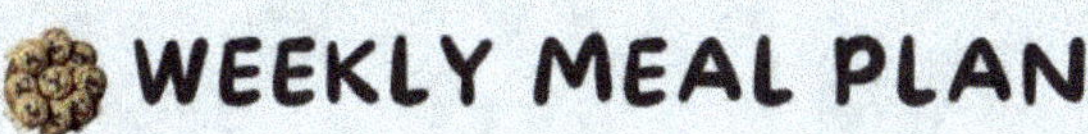

WEEKLY MEAL PLAN

MONDAY	
TUESDAY	
WEDNESDAY	
THURSDAY	
FRIDAY	
SATURDAY	
SUNDAY	

GROCERY LIST

FROM ________ TO ________

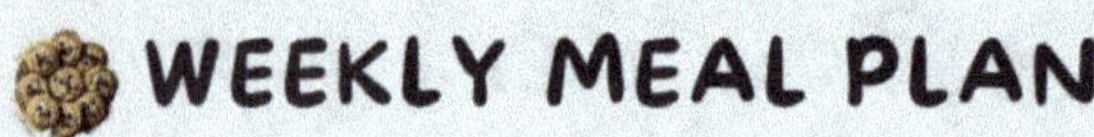 WEEKLY MEAL PLAN

		GROCERY LIST
MONDAY		
TUESDAY		
WEDNESDAY		
THURSDAY		
FRIDAY		
SATURDAY		
SUNDAY		

FROM _______ TO _______

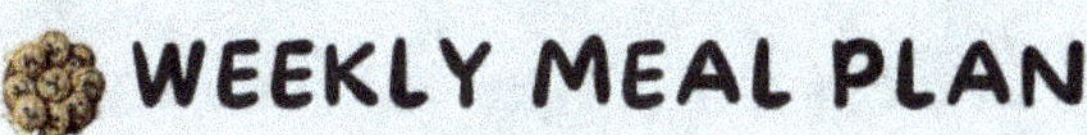 WEEKLY MEAL PLAN

	MONDAY
	TUESDAY
	WEDNESDAY
	THURSDAY
	FRIDAY
	SATURDAY
	SUNDAY

GROCERY LIST

FROM ________ TO ________

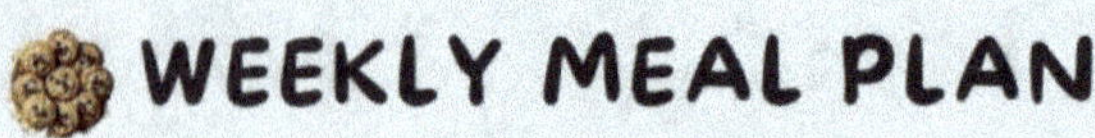

WEEKLY MEAL PLAN

MONDAY	
TUESDAY	
WEDNESDAY	
THURSDAY	
FRIDAY	
SATURDAY	
SUNDAY	

GROCERY LIST

FROM ________ TO ________

www.ingramcontent.com/pod-product-compliance
Lightning Source LLC
Chambersburg PA
CBHW061252250726
48653CB00002B/635